Food Rules for Weight Loss & Dieting

Perfect Health Begins with Perfect Food an End to Dieting

By: David Fry

Publishers Notes

Disclaimer

Digital Edition

What You Will Learn In This Book

How This Book Will Help You and Why

More and more persons are beginning to realize that food rules do help when it comes to maintaining the ideal weight and getting all the nutrients for the body to function properly. This book will outline how a diet should really be set up. It will also focus a bit on accelerated weight loss programs.

In addition to that the reader gets to learn about various diets and how they work, the 1000 calorie diet and the grapefruit diet are just two of the many that the author focuses on.

Dive Right into the Book! Or Learn a Bit More About the Author

TABLE OF CONTENTS

CHAPTER 1- DIETING THE HEALTHY WAY

Is it that you are having a tough time while following your diet plan? Is it that your dieting plans are failing constantly? Are you really adamant to make your diet plan work for you? Well as a matter of fact you should now acknowledge the truth that losing weight is an activity that does take time and there are no shortcuts to achieve weight loss. You need to keep this point in mind that a healthy eating plan begins with small steps. You can do the whole thing right but it does take a bit of time. However, if you begin making extreme changes and do not follow up with appropriate guidance then you are destined to go wrong. The following are some of the vital rules that will help you stick to your diet plant for good. This is actually dieting the healthy way.

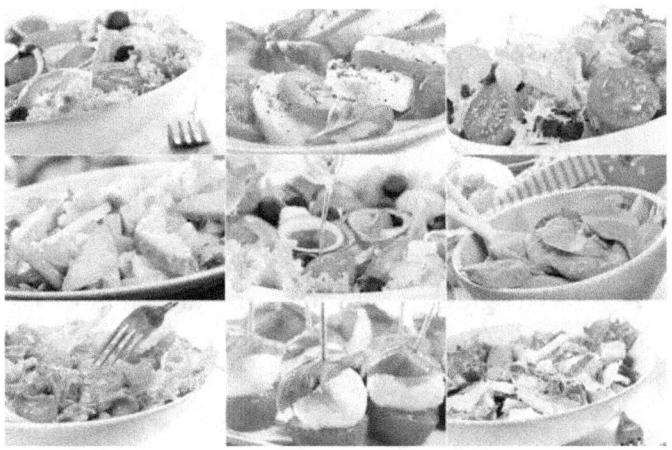

Find Ways To Eat Smartly: The choice of food items can be useful in reducing a lot of health related issues ranging from diabetes, heart problems and even cancer. You should be considering altering your diet plans as a set of stairs. You need to take your very first step and then take the rest. You should not be making drastic changes all at once but simple and easy adjustments initially. You should be starting out slow and keep making small alterations to your eating and consumption habits. This happens to be a general mistake most people make and one of the most prominent reasons why many people fail while considering making diet transformations.

Consider Lesser Portions: I am pretty much sure that you are well aware of how bite sizes have enlarged with the passage of time. Every individual wants to enjoy best value for the money they are spending and consequently portion sizes have been enlarged at various restaurants to realize the worth people have actually been probing for. This can turn out to be exceedingly dangerous to such people who are actually on a healthy diet. You may still prefer visiting a restaurant but you need to ensure that you are restricting your portions if you are eating half of your dinner and then save the rest for the next day's lunch.

Make Genuine Efforts: When you are aware of the fact that you cannot have something then you would certainly want it a lot more. It is a similar hypothesis of telling yourself not to fall down while you are on this stage, only to trip up over your own feet. You will be thinking about it energetically that you do not have to fall down or unintentionally encourage yourself not to be successful.

It's Not About What You Will Eat, But How You Will Eat: You possibly will eat just healthy diets but if you are consuming a large amount at one time, it is not going to do much good to you.

A healthy diet is a lot more in comparison to the food you have on your platter. Another key to triumph is how you actually think about various food items. You should never be rushing through your meals. You should slow down and eat with a calm and cool mind. This is because what you are eating is your requirement for nourishment and rushing it is not good for you. This is the time when you need to listen to your body, dining out with your friends and family is good but overdoing it is certainly not.

Hopefully I have been able to provide you with a considerable amount of information so that you can guide yourself while making your dieting plans and get started with an entirely new healthy eating diet lifestyle. In case you have come across a healthy eating diet program online, before you get started with it, you should be consulting your physician so that you can achieve your weight loss objectives.

CHAPTER 2- ACCELERATED WEIGHT LOSS PROGRAMS

There exist a multitude of diet plans to lose weight fast. Obviously, we live in a world where obesity and being overweight is extremely common. Most of the time, it's just a result of unhealthy diets like the Western diet which is loaded with useless calories.

In order to locate the best plan for you, you have to apply yourself. That means taking the time necessary to find what's been on the market, what's good, what's not and so on. It's called research. Try to avoid falling into traps set by advertisers who promised the world but never deliver. The most important thing is to choose a plan that will not have any negative impact on your health whatsoever.

Picking the right one comes from this research. And in your research, you must speak with your doctor. Furthermore, you can talk to your friends, family, and coworkers. Lots of people have been in this situation and can be helpful. They could tell you if something worked or didn't work. However, don't go buy something that they just heard. Make sure that they actually follow the plan themselves. Learn more about spinning back the scale to lose fat and shed pounds naturally.

Diet Plans To Lose Weight Fast

Sometimes you just need to lose a little bit of weight, and you need to lose it fast. Not everyone wants to wait around two or three months to drop those extra ten pounds, especially when they wanted it gone yesterday. That may be why so many diet plans to lose weight fast are around, almost ensuring at least one diet plan to lose weight fast will fit your weight loss needs.

The three-day regime is the perfect plan if you have less than ten pounds to shed. It is low calorie with a very easy meal plan. It consists of very basic foods with some substitutes like tuna instead of cottage cheese and green beans instead of broccoli for those who are not fans of certain healthy foods.

7 Day Diet Plan

The seven-day regime is one of those all-you-can-eat plans. However, the all-you-can-eat is limited to certain food groups at a time. An example of this is eating all the fruit you want, except bananas on Monday, and on Friday eating four 3-ounce pieces of beef, fish, or chicken with fresh vegetables throughout the day.

The Grapefruit Diet

The grapefruit diet has been around for decades, but despite its age, people still flock to it when they want to get rid of ten pounds fast. As the name suggest, grapefruit is used as it is believe that drinking or eating it with protein speeds up the fat burning process. This plan is very high in protein with eggs, bacon, and plenty of meat and is one of many diet plans to lose weight fast that really works. This diet will be discussed in greater detail in Chapter 6.

The Cabbage Soup Diet

The cabbage soup diet is another that has been around forever with a popularity that goes up and down. For seven days, you eat as much cabbage soup as you want mixed in with the daily fruit, vegetable, or meat you are allowed. The diet plans to lose weight fast eating cabbage comes with a recipe for the soup, which is mainly cabbage and some vegetables. It is said to work because you burn more calories eating cabbage than you ingest.

Chicken Soup Diet

Almost everyone has heard of diets for quick weight loss and the cabbage soup diet–with many hating it. Now another soup diet is making its rounds and it is much tastier, the chicken soup diet. This is a very simple idea; you eat one of the breakfasts offered in the plan, and then eat as much chicken soup as you want throughout the day. The soup does consist of a variety of vegetables, like carrots and broccoli, along with spices and of course chicken.

The Scarsdale Plan

For those that need to shed a bit more than just a few extra pounds, the Scarsdale plan is still popular. Created by a doctor of the same name, this is a very high protein regime that lasts for two weeks. There is no calorie counting and no measuring. The menu is simple yet not boring, and the menu has foods that fill you up and give you a boost of energy.

There are dozens and dozens of diet plans to lose weight fast today. Some are safer than others and some are harder than others are. Nevertheless, if you need to shed a few pounds quickly, you are sure to find diet plans to lose weight fast that work with your body.

Chapter 3- Low Carb Diet Tips

Are you overweight? Is your body obese? In case you answered yes to these two questions, surely you have to be looking for a solution to be fit, and rapidly. Mainly because these forms of weight reduction plans destroy muscle, the metabolism slows down. This is by no means a great factor and should not be utilized. Healthy diet plans will need to constantly be followed instead.

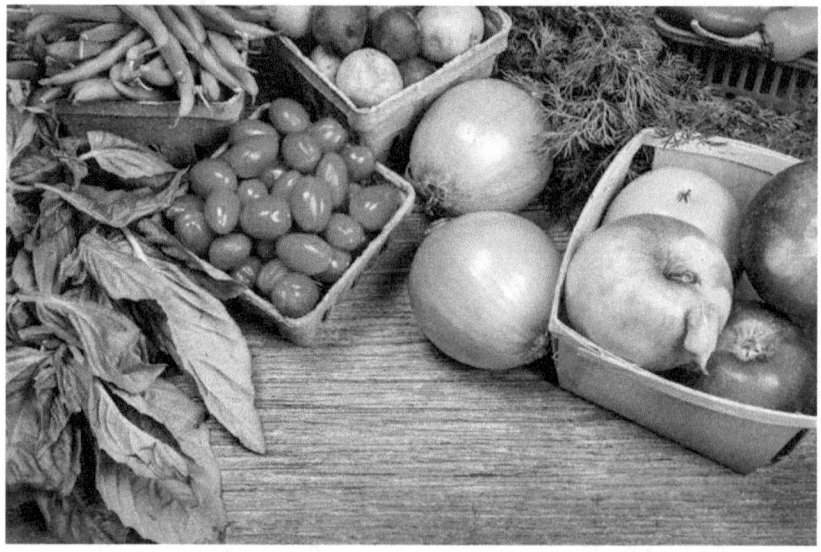

Let's commence with your nutrition plan. A habit of bad consuming practices invariably leads to excessive and unhealthy weight gain. Chances are, if you are not losing weight it is correlated to consuming bad foods. You have to have the discipline to follow a healthy diet plan to the end no matter what. Devoid of it, you may fail to have success even with most basic of diets.

Restrictive dieting plans are the antithesis of healthy diet plan plans. Restrictive eating only functions well in the short term. Individuals who eat this way will normally be forced to continue as a way to maintain their outcomes.

Weight-loss pills may perhaps claim to flush, block, or burn fat, and may well work to some extent, but most don't work at all. Scientists are still trying to locate methods to create this sort of pill. Some pills could be utilized to help control the appetite. Some, nonetheless, have severe side effects. Some could cause anxiety although others may trigger fatigue. Some of these pills are even addictive.

Plan meals in advance and place them in writing on the planner. Also let the youngsters get involved in the meal preparation stage as this is a superb time to educate them about nutrition, meal preparation and healthy foods. Healthy diet plans supply a substantially better approach.

People are becoming more carb conscious thanks to diets such as Atkins and South Beach. Carbohydrates get blamed for many people's weight problems. The truth is that not all carbs are bad. Good carbs do exist. After all, there is a reason athletes load up on carbohydrates before an event. The good carbohydrates give you energy. Despite what you may have read in an Atkins diet book, cutting out all carbohydrates is not healthy. The key to eating healthy is to eat a low amount of good carbs. Here are some tips on how to do that.

A low carb diet is usually associated with the idea that you get to eat lots of meat. That is one of the things that many people look forward to when they start low or no carb diets. Eating lots of meat is encouraged because most meats don't have carbohydrates. Beef, chicken, and seafood are all good meat choices on a low carb diet. This is the reason people on a low carb diet will substitute lettuce for the bun when eating a hamburger. This is good news for people who eat a lot of meat.

Many people think that eating lots of meat is the best part of following a low carb diet. While you can eat lots of meat, you shouldn't eat just any cut. While meat is free of carbs, it isn't free of fats or other unhealthy elements. Lean meats are your best choice when making your meals. The less fat on your meat dish the better you will be.

When following a low carb diet, cheese makes a great snack. Most cheeses do not contain carbs. Before chowing down, be sure to check the nutrition label. Some of cheeses, like feta, do contain small amounts of carbohydrates. If you want to use cheese as a healthy snack as part of a low carb diet, talk to your doctor or a nutritionist. The amount of carbs in the cheese is mostly dependent on how the cheese is made.

There are several ways to follow a low carb diet. It doesn't need to be a difficult process. You can feel full and still limit your carb intake by following these tips. Believe it or not, it is quite possible to live a very regular life while still making sure to keep your carb intake low. Eventually, the action that is now your conscious choice will become your habit. After a time, you won't even notice the difference anymore. You will only know that you feel better than you ever have.

CHAPTER 4- EASY WEIGHT LOSS TIPS

Diet has a huge impact on you losing those pounds. You can begin an effective weight loss plan by eating healthier and eliminating most of the junk food from your diet. You need to change both how and what you eat. For example, if you love to have mayonnaise and cheese on your white bread sandwich, simply cutting back on the mayo and cheese and changing your bread choice to whole wheat is a step in the right direction. This step needs to be included in all the food choices for your whole diet. Pay attention to what you are eating and ask yourself if it is a good, healthy choice.

Eat Your Veggies

Fruits and vegetables are highly recommended to help you lose weight. They are packed with fiber, antioxidants, vitamins, and minerals. Not only will they fill up your stomach and make you feel full, they are low in calories.

Make Simple Switches

Making just a few switches in the types of food you eat can greatly help you lose weight. As mentioned, replacing white bread with whole wheat bread is an easy weight loss tip for the extra fiber you will be adding to your diet. Fiber helps keep you fuller longer, hence fewer calories being consumed over the course of the day. Also, by trading in whole milk for non-fat or low-fat milk and replacing juice and soda with water, you can bet you will be shaving off calories and experiencing some rather easy weight loss. Another tip is instead of eating French fries, consider a baked potato, low-fat yogurt, or a salad with low-fat dressing.

What Not To Eat Or Drink

One tip for easy weight loss is to avoid certain foods. Soda pop is a great example as it can easily add up to 360 or more extra calories a day. Of course beer is another drink to avoid or limit while losing weight. You also want to avoid fast food, grease, and other junk food like chips and candy bars.

Eat Smaller Meals

When losing weight, cutting back on calories is essential. One way you can do this is by eating smaller portions. Another way is to avoid snacking or change what you nibble on. If you do need a snack, reach for apples and carrot sticks instead of chips and candy.

Drink Water

One of the best easy weight loss tips you will receive is to drink water. Water is a critical part of your diet, no matter what your weight. However, it is something most dieters overlook. You should drink a minimum of eight ounces a day. Drinking water will help your diet because it:

- Suppresses your appetite and helps you feel full so you will eat less

- Helps your metabolism run at its optimal rate
- Helps reduce fat deposits in your body
- Flushes out waste products as your fat cells are shrinking

Don't Remove All the Goodies

Keeping some treats in your diet may not seem like a tip for easy weight loss, but your sanity is important. Though junk food, sweets, and soda are not the best choices for you, you are only human. The best way to avoid ruining your diet is by rewarding yourself, in moderation. Allow yourself to eat something you really want that is unhealthy, but not on a daily basis. If you need a pop, have one on Friday evenings with dinner as a way to end the week. Keep those goodies in your life just enough so you will not feel like you are suffering. These little indulgences will help you stick to your otherwise healthy diet.

Exercise

Exercise, or be physically active, for 30 to 60 minutes a day. You can break this up into 15 minute blocks if you need to. However, you need to be moving or doing some fat burning and burning calories. Walking, aerobics, bike riding, jogging, jump roping, walking up stairs, or even playing with your Dance Revolution is exercise.

Set Small, Achievable Goals

Once you decide to lose weight, you need to set goals. Losing 30 pounds in a month is highly unlikely for anyone. Instead, focus on small, achievable goals. Start small. One to two pounds a week is a great starter goal. Another easy weight loss tip is to share your goal with others and ask them to hold you accountable. Find a friend or family member to share your progress with. Register at one of the many message boards dedicated to helping you lose weight. Having a buddy will help you stay on track.

Change Your Lifestyle

It will not do you any good to lose 15 pounds just to gain it all back. Often, we work so hard taking off the pounds that once we get there, we forget to work on maintaining our health. If you go back to your old eating and exercise (or lack of) habits as soon as you hit your goal, you will need to start all over again. So, while picking your diet program, make sure it is something you feel comfortable continuing for the rest of your life.

No matter how much weight you need to lose, it will not happen overnight. It involves creating good habits that will take time to develop.

CHAPTER 5- THE VEGETARIAN DIET

Switching to a healthy vegetarian diet might be motivated by the desire to wear your favorite jeans. However, in addition to a trim looking shape, other significant reasons exist to choose a new lifestyle. A healthy vegetarian diet is fresh, pure, alive, colorful, tasty, inviting, and prevents and fights disease. It has reduced fats with increased carbohydrates and fiber. It contains a multitude of vitamins, minerals, phytochemicals, and antioxidants. Finally, there is plenty of protein for infants, children, adults, and seniors. Every stage of life is appropriate to enjoy a healthy vegetarian diet.

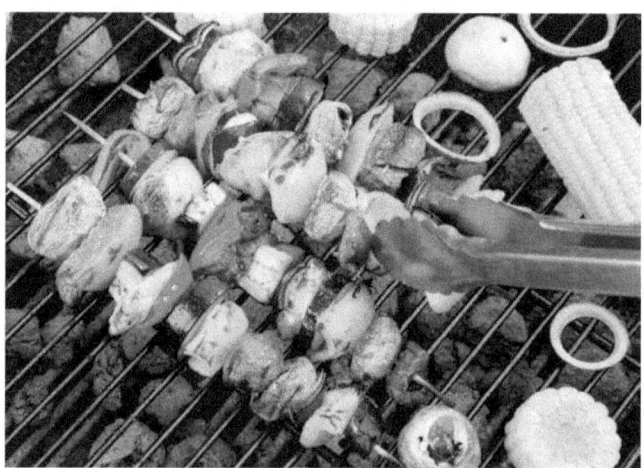

A few supplements should be considered when choosing a healthy vegetarian diet:

- Omega-3 is an essential fatty acid typically found in fish oil. One tablespoon of flax seed oil each day is the right amount of this nutrient.
- Vitamin B12 must be taken as a nutritional supplement due to the depleted condition of our soils. A cup of nonfat yogurt will meet B12 needs.
- To use calcium correctly requires Vitamin D, which doesn't necessarily have to be consumed. Fifteen to thirty minutes in the sun every couple of days" is all we need for our bodies to make the right amount of Vitamin D.
- Calcium is found in many healthy vegetarian diet foods. Look for dried herbs, sesame seeds (Tahini paste), tofu, almonds, flax seeds, green leafy vegetables (raw or cooked: spinach, turnip greens, kale, collards, mustard, dandelion greens, etc.), figs, white beans, Brazil nuts, and dairy items. Additionally, be sure to check packaged foods.

Look carefully at oatmeal, soymilk, rice milk and orange juice labels as they are often fortified with calcium.

Why Would I Choose A Healthy Vegetarian Diet?

- A healthy vegetarian diet heals the body and the soul; it always has.
- Hippocrates (460 – 357 BC), the father of medicine, is quoted as saying: He who does not know food, how can he understand the diseases of man?

- Dr. Campbell states "Fruits, vegetables and whole grains are the healthiest foods you can consume."
- Dr. Ox writes, "A complete carbohydrate-based diet that includes vegetables, legumes and beans, fruit, low-fat dairy, and soy products is advised."

What Diseases Can I Expect A Healthy Vegetarian Diet To Prevent Or Heal?

According to 750 research studies over 75 grant-years, a diet of meat, saturated fats, and sugars promotes the following diseases:

- Heart disease
- Cancer
- Obesity
- Diabetes
- Autoimmune disease
- Bone, kidney, eye and brain disease

Those same researches confirmed a low-fat, high carbohydrate diet based on plants and grains is the only way to prevent and/or reverse disease.

Can A Healthy Vegetarian Diet Prevent Or Reverse Heart Disease?

The more animal protein you eat, the more heart disease you will have. You can join 27.1 million Americans with heart disease. Plant protein dramatically lowers cholesterol levels more than reducing fat or cholesterol intake.

Can A Healthy Vegetarian Diet Prevent Or Reverse Cancer?

Research ongoing since 1946 discovered that countries with the highest healthy vegetarian diets had the lowest rates of cancer. Countries with the highest intake of animal protein had the highest rates of cancer. Clearly, eating healthier is preventive.

Cindy Nevills of Lakeland, Florida, had the diagnosis of Stage IV Melanoma in 2005. She changed to a healthy vegetarian diet. Her recent interview and picture of an able-bodied woman from a healthy vegetarian diet is dated February 2011.

Can A Healthy Vegetarian Diet Prevent Or Reverse Other Diseases?

Jason Wyrick was told in 2001 that he would be on medication his entire life due to a diagnosis of diabetes. He was not surprised, since diabetes runs in his family. He weighed over 330 pounds then. Today, he is trim and disease-free due to a vegetarian diet. Dr. Campbell's research shows that autoimmune, bone, kidney, eye, and brain diseases have all been prevented or reversed by a healthy vegetarian diet.

Don't wait. Begin your adventure toward health, self-confidence, happiness, and a disease-free lifestyle by eating a healthy vegetarian diet.

CHAPTER 6- THE GRAPEFRUIT JUICE DIET

The Grapefruit Juice Diet promises that in a period of two and a half months at most, you will lose approximately 15kilograms. By following some simple rules, you will have a body to envy. Be sure that your friends and colleagues will see the difference and will ask for your juicy secret.

Here are the "secrets" you should take into account when keeping the grapefruit juice diet:

- Drink at least two liters of water each day
- You can eat until saturation at each meal
- You must not eliminate any of the diet products; the mandatory products are ham and salads; these food combinations will burn your body fat, but if one of the products is eliminated, the diet won't work;
- Grapefruit juice has an important role in this diet, because it acts as a catalyst which begins by burning fat;
- do not reduce or add juice to this diet;
- You should give up coffee, because it affects the insulin balance and this will prevent burning fat; limit yourself to a cup per day at most;
- Don't eat between meals; if you only eat what we suggest you will not starve;
- You can fry food in butter and then use it for vegetables;
- Don't eat desserts, bread and white vegetables or sweet potatoes;

- You can double or triple your meat, salad and vegetable ratio ;
- You can eat until you feel full; the more you eat, the more kilograms you lose;
- Keep this diet for 12 days, have a two day break and restart it.

So, this is the diet plan:

Breakfast

- 250g of unsweetened grapefruit juice
- 2 eggs, cooked as you like;
- 2 slices of ham

Lunch

- 250g of unsweetened grapefruit juice
- Salad
- Any type of meat, in any quantity

Dinner

- 250g of unsweetened grapefruit juice
- Salad or green vegetables cooked in butter, or with spices
- Meat and fish, cooked as you like it
- Coffee or tea (one cup)

Bedtime Snack

- 1 glass of tomato juice or creamed milk

Here are other things you can consume : red onion, sweet pepper, radish, broccoli, cucumbers, carrots, green onion, spinach, cabbage, tomatoes, green beans, green salad, hot pepper, diet mayonnaise, any type of cheese, marinated vegetables, green vegetable, 1 spoon of dry peanuts, dill, bread.

The aliments you shouldn't consume are: white onion, potatoes, celery, peas, cereal, corn, vegetables from which you only consume the roots, peanut butter, pasta, potato and corn chips, jelly or jam, pretzels.

Chapter 7- The Pineapple Diet

According to recent research, the pineapple is considered one of the aliments which facilitate the process of burning fat, only by its simple consumption. How? It contains a substance, name bromeliad, which, besides its effect of burning fat, it also leads to the gradual disappearance of cellulite. Bromeliad is one of the few substances that are useful from the pineapple: besides it, there are a great number of minerals and vitamins, of which iron is the most important.

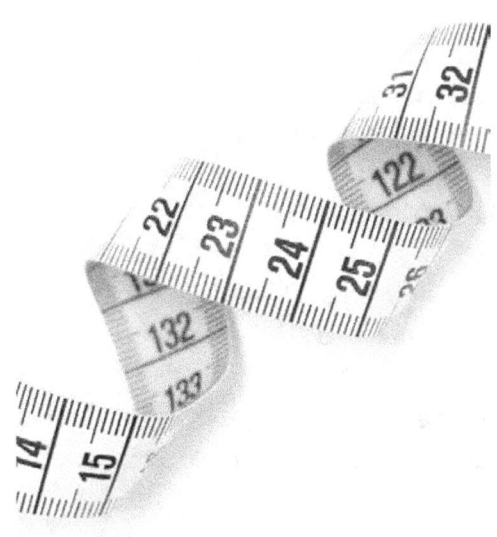

The pineapple diet is in the monodies category, which means it concentrates on the consumption of a single food in order to lose weight. Monodies are drastic forms of losing weight, that's why they are not recommended to be kept for more than ten days, or else they could deteriorate your well-being.

Diet Plan For Five Days

This plan lasts long enough for the process of detoxification to take place and for the loss of two to three kilograms, but it shouldn't be an extended diet.

- **Breakfast:** Two-three slices of pineapple and a Green tea (without sugar or with diet sweetener);
- **Snack:** A glass of pineapple juice (preferably, a home-made juice);
- **Lunch:** Vegetable soup and a piece of grilled fish or chicken;
- **Snack:** Pineapple juice and a pineapple low fat yogurt;
- **Dinner:** Five slices of pineapple.

Advantages of the pineapple diet:

- Helps with the rapid loss of weight;
- It contributes to the detoxification process of the organism;
- The cooked meals that you consume during the diet with pineapple are easily and rapidly made.

Disadvantages of the pineapple diet:

- It's a dull diet;
- During the diet with pineapple, your body doesn't retain as much liquids and it lacks a series of nutrients. That's why it's important to be careful with what you consume when you come back to your regular diet, because all the weight you have lost could easily be restored.
- The diet shouldn't be kept for a long time, because the pineapple doesn't ensure all the nutrients the body needs. Kept for long periods of time, the diet increases the risk of cardiovascular afflictions, renal problems and could even lead to muscle loss. Also, it can nurture anxiety and a general state of ill-being.

Pineapple Benefits

We all know that consuming a lot of fruits gives the body the daily necessary of antioxidants and vitamins. On top of that, each piece of consumed fruit could hold additional benefits, in some cases, even unique benefits.

Most people believe that calcium, dairy products, among which is milk, are primary elements which lead to the maintenance of strong and healthy bones. But, did you know that the pineapple contains manganese, an essential benefit mineral in the constitution of the conjunctive and bone tissue? A glass of pineapple juice contains approximately 73% of the daily requirement of manganese, which is recommended for healthy nourishment.

- **Coughs And Colds:** While the majority of people look for vitamin C supplements or orange juice when they feel a cold or a cough coming, most of them don't know that the best choice is the pineapple. The pineapple has not only the same components as the orange juice, but it also contains bromeliad, which acts upon the mucus and suppresses the cough.
- **Anti-inflammatory:** Are you suffering from osteoarthritis or joint pains? Because bromeliad is such an anti-inflammatory, you should consume at least half a glass of pineapple juice. It's a beneficent way to ease your pain.
- **Helps Digestion:** Another valuable benefit of the pineapple is that it contains the protheolitic enzyme, which, by definition, decomposes proteins. Thus, the pineapple helps the organism digest and efficiently use proteins.
- **Nausea In Pregnant Women:** The nausea can be difficult to bear for women with child. The consumption of fresh pineapple and nuts can reduce that state.
- **Reduces Allergies:** As research shows, consumed daily, these fruits reduce allergies and sinus related problems.
- **Reduces Blood Clots:** Another benefit of the pineapple is also known for the fact that it prevents the development of blood clots. Studies show that pineapple consumption can considerably reduce this risk.

Gives You A Boost Of Energy: The pineapple is an excellent manganese source, a co-factor for a great number for important enzymes in producing energy and anti-oxidant protection.

CHAPTER 8- THE 1000 CALORIE DIET

If you're currently looking for or considering going on a 1000 calorie diet then this just might be the most important thing you will read for a while. Scratch that, this will be the most important thing you read for a very long time because going on a low calorie diet is a mistake that many make and very few can ever rectify and this is simply because a low calorie diet and more specifically an 1000 calorie diet is going to do you no good whatsoever in the long run.

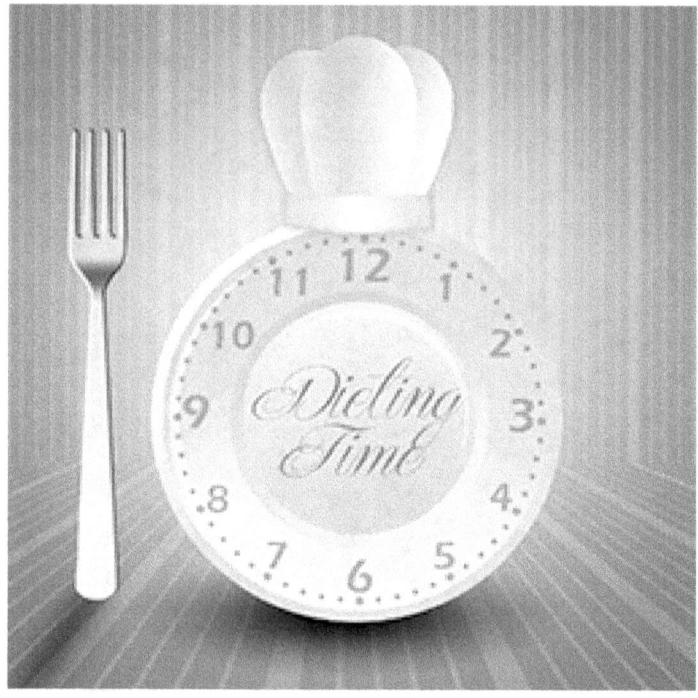

Now, to say that 1000 calorie diets do not work would be bending the truth a little bit because yes, you can lose weight with a low calorie diet but it is very difficult and more importantly, it is near impossible to keep the weight off when you've lost it with a low calorie diet.

The reason for this is simple; your body tries to burn the exact amount of calories you eat each and every day and gets into the habit of doing so.

So, when you first start your low calorie diet you will lose weight because you'll be eating significantly less and your body will be burning significantly more, no secret there. The problem arrives the second you decide that you've had enough of practically starving yourself and want to go back to eating a normal diet and this happens to everyone at some stage. Not only will you put all the weight you've worked hard on losing, you will pile on weight more than you ever have before.

Think about the reasons why you want to lose weight now. You're probably fed up of feeling low on confidence and want your self-esteem back. You probably don't like your appearance half as much as you would actually like and your health is nowhere near the level it should be.

It is harsh truth but one that you need to understand so that you don't fall for the traps of a low calorie diet because if you do, in a few months' time things will be significantly worse than they are right now.

Why people still feel as though low calorie diets are the answer, I have no idea. When you consider that low fat foods, low calorie foods and low carb diets have been around for years now and the state of obesity in society is only getting worse you can clearly see the flaws in how most people try to lose weight.

The weight loss industry is one of the biggest in the world and continues to grow year on year as people try to eat less. How many people are actually successful in their goal of losing weight? The answer is very few and if you don't want to fall into the failed dieter category then you need a weight loss solution that works and this is what I recommend.

Known as Fat Loss 4 Idiots, the program is designed to allow people who want to lose weight the chance to do so without having to starve themselves, spend hours a day at the gym or use a weight loss solution that is inevitably going to end by all that weight (and then some) being put back on in the end.

If you've dieted before or even attempted to lose weight through exercise then you will know first-hand that losing the weight is only half the battle, the other half is keeping the weight off and continuing to feel good about yourself every day.

Whilst low calorie diets, low fat foods, low carb diets and fasting don't work, Fat Loss 4 Idiots does and it has already serviced thousands of people around the world and been successful for all that have used it properly.

Using little known techniques to manipulate the fat burning hormones into working harder and faster, the Fat Loss 4 Idiots program allows you to lose around 9 pounds of weight every 11 days and this is one of the reasons it has become so popular.

There is nothing wrong with trying to lose a few pounds a week or losing weight slowly in theory but in reality it is not really a viable solution because weight loss takes an incredible amount of determination, motivation and willpower and many of us only have that drive to succeed for a few weeks before we resort back to bad, old habits. If you're losing weight quickly then that is not a big problem as in a few weeks from now you will be done and enjoying a vastly improved physique, sky high confidence and renewed self-esteem and just reading that must feel very, very good.

This is a method to losing weight that really works. Whilst you may have heard the "magic solution" sales pitch before, that is not really what Fat Loss 4 Idiots is offering. Sure, you may think that it is magic when you get inside the members and see all the little tips, secrets and techniques that have stopped you from losing weight in the past or will seriously accelerate your weight loss efforts but this in reality, is simply top quality information that you wouldn't necessarily know unless you were a professional in the health and nutrition market.

And perhaps best of all, there is nothing difficult about using Fat Loss 4 Idiots. The program is designed to help everyday people like you and I lose weight around our busy lifestyles, it will literally work for anyone. You've probably seen these "fad" diets that work for celebrities and yes they do work but the reason for that is their entourage of highly paid staff and ability to spend almost endless time in the gym.

For you and I that probably isn't an option and therefore something convenient is needed and Fat Loss 4 Idiots is it. Because all the methods used revolve around knowing what type of foods to eat in order to burn the most amount of weight you can easily get started today.

No need to spend another day feeling miserable about your weight, take action and start enjoying the "fruits" of weight loss with what I believe to be the best weight loss method on the market today.

Why 1000 Calorie Diets Don't Work

Have you ever wondered why following a 1000 calorie diet doesn't work as well as it should? One would think that practically starving yourself and eating so little vital calories would seriously help kick start the weight loss process and have you losing pound after pound in the blink of an eye. Unfortunately, the human body just doesn't work this way and following this low calorie diet is really just a recipe for disaster. Your body will be forced to function on little or no fuel, so your mind will be in a cloud all day long and you'll feel weak and fatigued while you are on this diet the entire time.

One reason why a 1000 calorie diet doesn't work is because the human body is easily capable of adapting to it, so it just doesn't stay that effective for a long period of time. This basically holds true for exercising as well. The longer you follow the same exercise routine, the less effective it is so you need to mix it up as much is possible if you want to see any signs of improvement. So following the same diet plan over and over will eventually become a routine that your body recognizes, and you will immediately hit a plateau because your body will only burn a certain amount of calories and then stop. This is a huge secret as to why low calorie diets just don't work, so you must vary your eating habits and vary your exercise routines if you ever truly want to see real gains that last as long as you want them to.

The other problem with following a 1000 calorie diet is that your metabolism will slow down a great deal once your body finally does adapt to this particular style of eating. Your metabolism will stay at the exact same level unless you begin to consume more calories or vary them one way or the other, although I don't recommend you lower your calories any further because you're already keeping them at a dangerous level to begin with. So certainly vary the amount of foods that you eat, and your metabolism will work at different speeds which will force it to work harder and burn fat quicker and properly.

When a person regularly consumes fewer calories by following a 1000 calorie diet, this forces you to consume less of the vital building blocks that keep a body functioning properly. You'll be eating less of the essential fats that are needed for healthy functioning, and diets like this also tell you to cut back on your intake of water which is also obviously a very essential part of healthy living and having a quality lifestyle that you can enjoy.

Instead of following a 1000 calorie diet, you should choose to eat healthy and smart instead. I recommend that you eat six times a day instead of the normal three that is usually recommended. This way your body will have fuel to allow you to function throughout the day, but you'll be eating small portions so you won't overdo it at any point and you'll burn the fat that you're trying to lose.

The Danger Of The 1000 Calorie Diet

There are plenty of reasons to want to give a 1000 calorie diet a shot, but most people don't have any real clue that a diet like this is actually very dangerous and it can seriously harm you instead of put you back on the road to good health which is what you're really trying to achieve anyway. There are some serious potential side effects that you might experience, and you can unfortunately put your long-term health at risk when you limit your calories to such a low level. So please take a look at the five risk factors that you really need to keep away from in order to avoid the dangers of a 1000 calorie diet.

The first big risk I'd like to mention regarding a 1000 calorie diet is dehydration. You probably don't realize that restricting your calories like this is going to cause you to lose weight rapidly, but the majority of the weight that you are actually losing is water weight. You must drink at least 1 gallon of water a day if you want to avoid dehydration and continue to stay healthy.

Feeling tremendous amounts of fatigue on a 1000 calorie diet is often a major complaint from those who are following a diet such as this. If you seriously limit the fuel that your body can use, then you can expect to function at a much lower level. So you'll definitely feel a lot more tired since you don't have the right amount of fuel in your system needed to function on a day-to-day basis. This will cause you to experience a lot less energy, so only do light exercising if you insist on following a dangerous diet plan such as this.

The other major danger that people aren't aware of when following a 1000 calorie diet is that they seriously slow down their metabolism. Your body will switch into survival mode and intentionally lower your metabolism because limiting your calories tricks your body into believing that it needs to store fat for fuel because a famine is on the way. This dates back to the beginning of time when man would often experience long periods without having any food to eat. We haven't evolved past this yet so consuming few calories will actually hurt your chances of losing weight.

The fourth danger of a 1000 calorie diet that really needs to be mentioned is malnutrition. By eating so few calories you will obviously be subjecting yourself to an unbalanced diet and a meal plan that really is improper for anyone. This is just way too few calories for the human body to function properly, so you are putting yourself at risk of becoming very unhealthy due to the lack of the proper nutrients your body needs in order to thrive and survive.

The final danger that I'd like to mention of a 1000 calorie diet is the higher likelihood that you will gain back all the weight once your diet is over. You're much better off going on a diet that shows you how to eat healthily and maintain a normal weight, because finishing a diet like this usually means you go back to your normal eating habits and you'll immediately begin to pack on the pounds as soon as the diet is over. There's no point suffering through all of that if you're only going to immediately gain all the weight back again.

About The Author

David Fry was not always healthy. At age sixteen he was a whopping three hundred pounds and had quite a number of health problems. He had tried numerous diets and barely lost any weight. In a last bid effort he was ready to do gastric bypass surgery to see if that would help him to shed the weight. His doctor asked him to try one last thing before he opted for the surgery. He sent him to a nutritionist to restructure his diet.

David was opposed to this at first as he had seen nutritionists before but decided to try it anyway. It was slow going at first and he was frustrated but with encouragement and support he stuck to it. After abiding to the food rules and incorporating exercise he soon found that he was shedding those extra pounds. His experience led to him writing about food rules.

www.ingramcontent.com/pod-product-compliance
Lightning Source LLC
Chambersburg PA
CBHW060442290526
45793CB00002B/536